INSIGHTS

an imprint of

INSIGHT EDITIONS

www.insighteditions.com

MANUFACTURED IN CHINA

10 9 8 7 6 5 4 3 2 1